WHO[...]
CANCER
THERAPY

- Hyperthermia
- Laetrile
- Oncotox
- Germanium
- Ozone
- Interferon
- Flutamide
- Beta-Carotene
- Carbatine
- Visualization

- Hydrogen Peroxide
- Clodronate
- Hydrazine Sulfate
- Bio-Magnetics
- Thymus Therapy
- DMSO
- Thymus Extract
- Live Cell Therapy
- Shark Cartilage
- Drip of Life

© 1993

Kurt W. Donsbach, D.C., N.D., Ph.D.
H. Rudolph Alsleben, M.D., D.O., Ph.D.

Table of Contents

Wholistic Cancer Therapy

Cancer is one of the most common causes of death in the United States and the most feared of all diseases. By their own statistics, medicine and research have not made any progress in the treatment of cancer since the 1950's. In fact, some of the cancers are more prevalent today than they were back then. This is a serious indictment of our medical system which has cried "wolf" for so long in order to raise billions of dollars to research this dread disease. Fat grants have not found the cause, much less the cure. After years of denial, the National Cancer Institute has finally agreed with the vocal minority of nutritionists that diet is related to cancer. But, they steadfastly deny the many successful alternative therapies which are available in various parts of the world.

This booklet is a compilation of the therapies which are actively employed at Hospital Santa Monica, located on beautiful Santa Monica Beach, just north of Rosarito Beach on the Baja coast of Mexico. We have spent most of our adult lives practicing, researching, writing and teaching (some have called it preaching) the gospel of good nutrition. During that time, we have had the honor and privilege of knowing, sharing and learning from some of the most innovative healers in the world. Some of them were medical doctors, chiropractors, naturopaths, osteopaths and dentists; while others professed to be successful with techniques that were not licensed or generally accepted. "One should walk in another's shoes for three moons before judging." The wisdom in that statement was brought out many time as we learned that when one took the time to understand what the "quack remedy" was all about, one found that indeed there was a basis for the theory.

Modern day medicine would have us believe that the "consensus of medical opinion" is the final criteria for judging any and all approaches to health. Talk about the fox watching the chicken coop! This is like asking a fundamentalist preacher to judge the eastern religions. There is so much "brainwashing" going on in the many years of schooling that medics go through, it is impossible for them to look with an unjaundiced eye upon any healing art other than their own, which is, of course, the only true one.

In no field of medicine is there more rigid control of the patient than in the treatment of cancer. Surgery, chemotherapy and radiation are the only accepted modes of therapy which a physician may use without being censored by his peers. Attempts by doctors to use innovative therapies, even with terminal patients without any hope, have met with swift and efficient ejection from the profession.

This is so unfair and immoral that I have always found it difficult to understand why individuals who live in a (free) society allow their legislators to continue to pass laws which actually take away a citizen's freedom to choose how their body will be treated if they are ill. One of these days, an aroused citizenry will rise against these illegal bonds and demand (as the chiropractors did) that federal law inhibit a single branch of the healing arts from monopolizing all healing.

It has been out of experience that the diagnosis of cancer is not the "kiss of death." Unfortunately, the alternative or wholistic practitioner only sees the patient after all else has failed - surgery, chemotherapy and radiation. It is when the final words, "We can do no more," are uttered by the same physician who said, "We got it all," that patients begin to look for a ray of hope. It is a miracle that any of these patients survive - but amazingly, a majority do. The feeling of victory that comes when a patient leaves the hospital on a definite upswing, feeling better and free of pain with blood tests indicating fast improvement, is impossible to describe.

The treatments and medicines which will be described in this booklet are not the wishful thinking of a self-appointed savior. They have been widely researched in various countries of the world; but for one reason or another, they have not been "blessed" by the Food and Drug Administration for use in terminal patients in the United States.

Some very esteemed personalities have pointed out that hope sometimes can be responsible for a total reversal of an irreversible disease. So this booklet is about hope - based upon legitimate research and personal experience. The last 4 years have been the most significant and possibly the culmination of years of soaking up wisdom from whatever sources we could find.

Hospital Santa Monica is the largest truly Wholistic hospital in the world. To have this facility and the opportunity to offer what we believe in is the fulfillment of our fondest dream.

REASONS I BELIEVE - KWD

I have been charged many times for professing that unknown and unproven remedies are effective in the treatment of "incurable" diseases. Such charges are always levied by governmental agencies which are backed by willing experts to testify that the substance has never been properly tested or published in a "legitimate" medical journal. Since the procedure for testing costs a minimum of 50 million dollars and will usually take up to 10 years, the pharmaceutical industry wants a product that will eventually return a lot of money before they make the investment.

The products I have been working with are usually non-proprietary and cannot be protected. Thus the possibility of such research and testing ever occurring is dim indeed. All of this need for research and testing of non-proprietary and non-toxic remedies is due to the FDA ruling that "any substance used for the treatment, prevention, cure or mitigation of disease (and a long list is given) shall be considered a drug." The interpretation of this is that if you use cabbage juice for the treatment of an ulcer, cabbage is a drug. Or Vitamin E for heart disease or water for constipation, etc. This can become ridiculous, as you can easily see.

CLINICAL EVIDENCE

My position on these various substances comes from clinical observations, in other words, patients responding. Recently I have been charged with saying that hydrogen peroxide is of benefit in the treatment of an incurable disease, namely arthritis and as a treatment for cancer. If such is a crime, then I have to plead guilty. I sincerely believe that I have freedom of the press and freedom of speech to report what I believe. It may take a court to judge this.

Regardless, here are some of the reasons I speak and write as I do. I cannot morally keep such news to myself.

This is a letter from a 26 year old patient with an incurable disease, according to his doctors. I believe his story is pertinent.

Quote:
April 20, 1988
RE: Case History of Michael Jones, Psoriatic Arthritis Patient.

In November 1983, a rash began to appear on my head, accompanied by great amounts of dandruff. After an attempt to control this problem with products found on drug store shelves, scaling began to appear. Seeking relief from the itching and flaking, I began seeing dermatologists; they diagnosed by problem as psoriasis. These doctors prescribed steroid creams and special shampoos that cost a fortune. After one year, I still had not found any relief and the psoriasis continued to spread.

In October 1986, I began to experience pain in my toes that would last for short periods of time. As weeks passed, the pain continued to increase until was I was in constant pain.

At times, my toes would swell so large that the joints felt like they would burst. In May 1987, doctors diagnosed my problem as psoriatic arthritis. They treated this condition with drugs such as Feldrene and Motrin (in large amounts) which were also very expensive and provided little relief. I began to substitute arthritis-strength aspirin for the Feldrene and Motrin and was taking approximately 30 tablets per day.

The arthritis and psoriasis continued to deteriorate and began to move into the upper part of my body. By September 1987, I began using a cane to help me walk 90% of the time. I went from working 12-15 hour days to being able to work only 2-4 hours a day. On rainy or cold days, I was almost immobile with pain. I became very dependent on my wife, she would rub arthritis pain relief ointments on me at night. She also had to help me bathe, dry off (I could not reach the lower part of my body, especially my toes), help me get in and out of the tub (or I would fall), and help me get dressed.

A friend of mine began telling me about the use of hydrogen peroxide in the relief of these types of diseases. We began to search for information regarding this type of treatment and found ECHO, an organization dedicated to the research of hydrogen peroxide. Among the information provided by ECHO was a reference about a clinic run by Dr. Kurt Donsbach in Rosarito Beach, Mexico. There was a phone number for this clinic so I contacted Dr. Donsbach's office and asked for information. They sent me a video tape of Hospital Santa Monica showing the facilities and interviews with some people who had been helped by Dr. Donsbach. After careful consideration, my wife and I decided to give Dr. Donsbach a try.

My wife and I left Atlanta on January 19, 1988 and arrived in San Diego the same day. We were met at the airport and taken to the hospital without any problems at all. The evening we arrived, I was given an entrance examination (including blood and urine test) and was interviewed by several doctors and Dr. Donsbach. After these meetings, a plan of treatment was laid out consisting of hydrogen peroxide infusions, colonics, massages, reflexology, hydrogen peroxide whirlpools, intramuscular shots and a proper diet including vitamins and supplements. I began my treatment the next day; that night, after my hydrogen peroxide infusion, I developed a bad headache and began to get very ill. The next morning my skin had turned cherry red. Dr. Donsbach explained that this was toxins leaving my body. I became very ill and consequently spent the next four days and nights in bed.

On the fifth day, I began feeling much better and found that upon arising, I didn't need my cane to help me walk, or the assistance of my wife to help me bathe, dry myself, and get dressed. As each day passed, greater progress was achieved. I could walk a little farther and get a little more exercise each and every day. By the end of the second week, I could ride the bicycle in the exercise room for two miles on the middle setting. At the end of the third week, I was riding the exercise bicycle 3.5 miles and day and taking a daily walk on the beach. At the time of this letter, I have now worked my way up to 10 miles on the uphill setting and continue to feel better every day.

Dr. Donsbach and Hospital Santa Monica have my support in the treatments provided for arthritis. Anyone who has questions or would like to discuss this further with me, please feel free to call. I am excited about my recovery and would like to see others receive relief from the same horrible pain that I once experienced. I am indebted to the staff of Hospital Santa Monica and Dr. Donsbach for returning my health and my life back to me. I am sure that without their help, I would now be an invalid and confined to my home.

(Signed) Michael D. Jones
Unquote (tel. on file)

Letters such as this and the witnessing of so many others who also had results make it very difficult to not share with those in pain. Here is one on the subject of cancer.

Quote
April 18, 1988
Dear Friends,

I am, or should I say was, a 43 year old terminal breast cancer patient. Last fall, my doctor patted me on the back and sent me home to die. Oh, they suggested more radiation and chemotherapy, but I refused, having already had one unsuccessful go-round with "burning and poisoning" that had left me bald.

After going through lumpectomy, removal of underarm lymph nodes, two biopsies, and finally mastectomy, which included skin grafts from both legs, the cancer was once again creeping over my entire chest and invading my one remaining breast.

I had been on a strict natural diet for more than a year, but it just wasn't enough by itself. I needed something more, something stronger but without side-effects. I was out of options when one of "God's Messengers" handed my husband some literature on the hydrogen peroxide therapy.

I have just returned from a three week stay at Hospital Santa Monica in Mexico where this treatment is being given. My first week there, I slept most of the time, but after just ten days, I began to notice an improvement on my chest and was soon up exchanging mutual support with the other patients.

I also had a lump under my arm the size of a quarter

which had gone down to half that size by the time my stay was up. I also witnessed many other sufferings being eased during my visit. I saw a man come in on a stretcher with a brain tumor who was up serving himself in the dining room ten days later.

While I am not yet cured, my cancer has definitely been arrested and is continuing to fade away daily. When I look back at all I have been through, I realize I will never be quite the same person I was, as my stay at the Hospital was a spiritual experience as well as a physical one for me.

I will be eternally grateful to the staff at the Hospital, but I can't be more content in my heart at just leaving it at that. I want to make it my duty to spread the word. For those who have nowhere else to turn, let it be known that there is a choice. Give alternative therapy a chance! God Bless You All.

(Signed) Naomi Thomas
Unquote

HYPERTHERMIA

The traditional methods for treating cancer are surgery, chemotherapy and radiation. Because the survival rate is poor and the body is subjected to toxic and damaging effects of the therapies, an alternative has been sought by therapists worldwide.

12

Investigation of the world's literature reveals a number of non-toxic, natural/nutritional therapeutic approaches that have impressive tumor reduction and life improvement capabilities. We have assembled the best of the "alternative" methods available globally into a therapy program which has been used at our hospitals in Mexico and Poland for over 12 cumulative years. We call our protocol the AL-DON METHOD.

Our research division, the Al-Don Medical Research Institute, is in constant computer contact with several global medical research data-bank libraries. As new therapies are developed and tested by the finest medical institutions in the world, we are able to include them in our hospital protocols long before they are available through traditional medical centers. The latest addition to our arsenal of wholistic cancer therapies is an innovative and improved version of microwave hyperthermia.

PULSE MODULATED MICROWAVE HYPERTHERMIA™

Pulse Modulated Microwave Hyperthermia, the Al-Don microwave method developed by Drs. Donsbach and Alsleben, in conjunction with Cheung Laboratories, kills or damages cancer cells, starves cancer cells and helps to poison cancer cells without damaging normal tissue.

We have the first and only pulse modulated microwave hyperthermia unit the world. With PM Microwave Hyperthermia, three dramatic therapeutic benefits are possible: 1. Exposure of tumor tissue to 915 megH. frequencies and wave forms; 2. Thermal heating of tumor tissue to cancer cell critical temperatures; 3. Micro-transmission of neural-healing encoded instructions to assist in tumor regression.

Controlled PM Microwave exposure of a tumor has proved to be very effective in not only destroying or reducing tumor mass, but also undermining the cancer cell's ability to survive, resist immune assault and obtain adequate nourishment. Microwave heating of the tumor mass is accomplished by very sophisticated instruments which monitor the energy delivered to the tumor cells. Tumor hyperthermia, increased heat in the tumor, is accomplished by directing a carefully controlled microwave beam of energy into the mass of the tumor to increase its temperature to the bio-critical level. At this temperature, a number of things happen to the cancer cells which affect their viability. To understand these effects, we must discover how cancer cells are born, how they reproduce and obtain nourishment, and how they resist attack by the immune system, chemo-therapeutic drugs and radiation.

HOW ARE CANCER CELLS BORN?

1. Cancer cells can be compared to orderly citizens who have suddenly become disorderly. They seem to evolve without regard to the rules by which normal cells live and grow. The effect may be genetic in that the genetic code may have an instruction to produce a cancer cell, or something normal within the code may have been

modified to become abnormal.

2. Cancer cells may come about as a result of chemical or electromagnetic damage to a normal cell which, short of killing it, caused it to become cancerous.

3. Cancer cells may come about as a result of a normal cell changing its characteristics in response to an alien agent, chemical, virus, bacteria, fungus, mold or nerve transmission.

Pulse Modulated Microwave Hyperthermia is our most dramatic physical modality to induce tumor regression and cancer cell destruction. As cells (both normal and cancerous) multiply, they require more nourishment that only blood can provide. All tissue cells contain instructions within their genetic code that stimulate the growth of new blood vessels to supply their accelerated growth. Cancer cells have a deranged instructional pattern or blueprint for making new blood vessels which causes the new vessels to be defective. This results in inadequate and inefficient blood supply to the rapidly expanding growth. Heating tissue, whether in normal or cancerous tissue, causes the cells to increase their metabolic rate. An increased metabolism results in an increased demand for nourishment and an increased population of waste products. Normal tissues are able to obtain adequate nourishment and detoxification because they have an adequate and competent blood and lymph supply. Cancer tissue has an inadequate and incompetent blood and lymph supply, therefore, nourishment and detoxification are impeded. The cancer cells starve at the same time they undergo a self-induced toxic self-destruction. In the process of losing their grip on life, they become more susceptible to immune system attack, chemotherapy, radiation and specific nutrient factors which can create a more normal environment not compatible with tumor growth.

It is known that blood flow increases with the application of heat. When normal tissue is heated by microwave hyperthermia, the blood flow can increase by a factor of ten, whereas tumor circulation increases by a factor of only one or two. When microthermal heating (applied for 30-60 minutes) is stopped in normal tissue, the blood flow returns to the pre-treatment normal very quickly. In tumors, the blood flow falls far below what it was before treatment. This results in continued and rapid starvation of the tumor cells while there is no adverse effect on normal tissue. Cancer cells require huge amounts of energy which they obtain largely from glucose sugars in the body. The reduced blood flow reduces the available fuel energy, thereby starving the cancer cells.

We have capitalized upon this factor by utilizing substances which selectively block the tumor cell's ability to metabolize glucose. These formulas, developed by Dr. Donsbach, are carried to the target cells by cellular trophic (carrier molecule) nutrients so that the cancer cells are further starved for energy. With their energy supply and structural integrity disrupted, the cancer cells have less resistance to immune system attack and the tumor repressive effects of specific nutrients.

Another important factor concerns information going to the tissues and cells via nerve fibers. Nerve impulses give instructions to the cells that control their metabolism and permeability which determine metabolic functions, rate, resistance and porosity of the cell wall. Permeability changes control the intake of nutrients and output of toxins. Cancer cells are "renegades." They are not connected to the intelligence network of the nervous system. They operate completely on their internal genetically programmed "instinct." Could cancer cells be brought under better control if they received normal nerve instructions? Microwaves can transmit normal neural intelligence if it is properly encoded into frequency patterns which they can carry. Unlike other instruments, our microwave generators have devices attached to them that can transmit normal brain wave and specific laser frequencies into the tumor to modulate cancer cell functions.

Finally, it is well known that certain viruses, bacteria and fungi are associated with tumor production and growth. These dangerous and destructive microbes are rendered ineffective, damaged or dead by microwave energy when the temperature reaches the cancer cell bio-critical temperature.

In summary, pulse modulated microwave hyperthermia is a very dynamic, corrective therapy for many cancers. When added to the wholistic programs in the Al-Don Method, the results can be astonishing.

Our microwave instruments are specially designed to

function completely on the outside of the body. Sophisticated energy control computer programs measure and monitor the precise temperatures being generated. The equipment has built-in, fail-safe energy control circuit breakers which prevent temperatures harmful to normal tissues.

IMMUNE MODULATOR BLUEPRINTS

Another major breakthrough in cancer patient management is the Al-Don Immune Modulator Blueprints. Current medical literature indicates that up to 90% of cancers are caused by environmental factors such as pollution, toxic chemicals, asbestos, airborne particulate matter, industrial chemicals in the air, water and food, electromagnetic radiation, trauma, dyes and stains. The list is endless. It is now well established that certain viruses, fungi, molds and bacteria are implicated in the production of cancer. Vaccines have already been produced against some of these microbes and their effect can be quite astonishing.

The Al-Don Method includes "immune modulator blueprints," an improvement upon the autogenous and heterogenous vaccine concept produced by Drs. Virginia Livingston, von Brehmer and Enderlein for members of the family of microbes related to disease and tumor production. We have improved upon the vaccine concept by including immune modulators for the microbial life cycles before and after the stages implicated in tumor growth. We believe that our Tri-Vac Immune Modulator Blueprints lead the field in cancer immunology.

Our philosophy, and the core of the effectiveness of the Al-Don Method, is to constantly improve the quality and applicability of our treatment programs. Several of the outstanding physicians in the history of the fight against disease have discovered micro-organisms related to disease production. Such discoveries were possible only because those scientists were sufficiently brave and creative to look for new explanations. New microbes have been discovered.

New theories about the origins of these microbes have been hypothecated. Al-Don research has found a breakthrough explanation for the origin of bacteria and fungi related to diseases, such as cancer, and the reason for metastases of cancerous tumors. With these new research findings, we are developing technologies capable of treating cancerous growths before they occur: in other words, disrupting the usual malignant-metastatic pathway.

THE ROLE OF THE IMMUNE SYSTEM

We must acknowledge that viruses, bacteria, parasites and genetic causes for cancer have always been here and yet more cases of cancer are being reported every year. Just think of it, a million people with cancer die in this country every year (and most of them die in spite of all available therapy). Cancer is now the second leading cause of death in young people. Many of the causative agents have been here since the beginning of man, yet the number of cases increases every year at an out-of-control epidemic rate. How did mankind survive to this

19

day? Mankind survived because of his immune system. A competent immune system adequately kills the newly-developing cancer cells before they become a tumor. If the immune system is not competent, cancer cells, bacteria, fungi, molds and viruses are allowed to flourish and further undermine the body's resistance to diseases of all kinds.

Our wholistic protocols include a number of therapies capable of restoring the immune system to normal function.

SUMMARY

The Al-Don Method is a comprehensive, alternative, wholistic therapy program consisting of many of the world's most effective, non-toxic therapies. The intensive, well-balanced therapy protocol is delivered during a 14 day stay at either of our hospitals.

QUESTIONS ABOUT MICROWAVE

Q: Are microwaves dangerous?

A: Is sunlight dangerous? Is water dangerous? The answers are obviously yes and no! Yes, if there is too much. No, if there is too little. Microwaves are in the radio portion of the electromagnetic spectrum. Microwave exposure of certain frequencies, at certain power levels, over certain periods of time can be dangerous. Medical microwave frequencies are more healing than destructive. They are not scattered to affect the entire body, they are focused and isolated to affect only a small portion of the body for a relatively short time, specifically the tumor. Generally speaking, the frequency of our microwave therapy is beneficial in that it promotes healing and the immune response. Special forced air and air cooled applicators have been developed by Cheung Laboratories to isolate the microwave energy into a narrow beam which can be directed specifically to the tumor while insuring that skin temperatures stay well within tolerable levels.

Q: Can the microwaves "cook" the tumor?

A: Not the way we use them. We have three objectives in our microwave therapy sessions. 1. To deliver the 915 megH frequency beam into the tumor area. 2. To heat the tumor tissue up to as high as 42 degrees centigrade (non-toxic to normal tissue). 3. To transmit neural frequency instructions into the tumor. "Cooking" the tumor is not necessary nor even desirable. It is far more effective to injure the tumor than it is to kill it. By injuring the tumor, your body can gradually dissolve and eliminate its debris safely.

Q: When can results be observed?

A: In surface tumors, changes may be detected immediately or may take several days. The speed of alteration is not important. It is what happens to the tumor in the long run that is important. We prefer the changes to be gradual so that the body can resorb and detoxify at its own speed and capability. We plan our programs so that adequate time is allowed for our wholistic therapies to begin health restoration. A sick body is less capable of detoxification than a well body. To our knowledge, we are the only hospital in the world to combine an extensive wholistic therapy program with hyperthermia, which is why our results are so gratifying.

Q: Is it necessary to pinpoint the tumor location in order to use microwave hyperthermia?

A: This is also a yes and no answer. 1. If thermal heating of the tumor mass is the primary application of the microwave energy, then the tumor should be approximately located and be within the energy penetration range. The microwave applicator antenna transmits a beam of sufficient diameter to have a "shotgun" coverage of the tumor site. This is especially true if the tumor is quite large. A second advantage to our particular microwave equipment is that it has two antenna applicators which can be used simultaneously for greater area coverage if needed or to energize two different tumors at the same time. Remember that physicians have considerable knowledge of the internal anatomy of the human being. If microwave therapy is being considered as an option for therapy, it would be helpful for patients to bring whatever examination records, especially x-rays and scans with them. It is our policy to perform non-harmful ultrasound scans of the appropriate body zones to localize known tumors and explore for unknown lesions. X-ray examinations are performed if necessary. 2. If the primary objective is frequency exposure of the tumor site rather than thermal generation, then the precise location of the tumor, especially if it is very small, is less critical. There are two categories of microwave experts in the world. Those who believe that the frequency is more important than the heat generated, and those who believe that the heat generated is more important than the frequency. Rather than go to the right or left of the truth, we prefer to take the middle path and seek both benefits. Much research is underway worldwide to understand the mechanisms for the healing effects of the 915 megH energy frequency. Our studies indicate that an immune enhancement is obtainable no matter where the beam is applied. For example, it is known that certain wavelengths of the ultraviolet electromagnetic spectrum, when exposed to the skin, inhibit the activity of the T-lymphocyte division of the immune system in the exposure site. It is also known that wherever the exposure is made, the entire lymphocyte population of the body can be effected. We believe that certain microwave frequencies have this same potential. It is for this reason that we are willing to expose "hard to hit" tumor regions, even though some physicists will argue that the beam cannot heat to those levels.

Q: How much heat is generated in tissue exposed to microwave energy and what temperatures are most effective?

A: In the early days of microwave generators and therapy protocols, frequencies were much lower and were able to penetrate deeper and heat to higher temperatures. The advantage to the lower frequencies was that deep tumors could literally be "fried." The disadvantages were that a totally destroyed tumor became a dangerous burden for the detoxification systems and the tissues between the skin and the tumor were frequently damaged. The older technologies required the surgical placement of temperature sensing probes within the tumor, a procedure not without risk. We rejected the microwave units that performed in that manner and waited instead for the most recent development of the 915 megH frequency generators with computer modulated temperature controls that did not require invasive temperature sensing probes or intermediate tissue damage. It can be said with reasonable certainty that the latest generation of microwave generators are <u>safe and fool-proof</u>. An additional safety factor with our equipment is that we see the maximum power output and temperature generation before the treatment starts. If, at any time during the therapy, the power or temperature inadvertently goes beyond our desires, the instrument automatically shuts off. It is known that cancer cells undergo substantial damage if they are heated to 104-108 degrees Fahrenheit while normal cells are unaffected. We see no need to go beyond that level.

Q: Is microwave therapy beneficial in cancer therapy if used by itself?

A: This is a good question. The answer is definitely yes. However, we have no intention of stopping at the second or third best position. We strive for maximum benefit by combining our microwave therapy with all of our wholistic and nutritional programs. For example, through careful and painstaking research, we have discovered natural substances which can block the cancer cells ability to obtain food. When cancer cells are starved and attacked by an aroused and nourished immune system at the same time that they are damaged, the result is far better. Most traditional hospitals and clinics using microwaves hyperthermia tend to combine it with radiation and chemo-therapy rather than wholistic approaches. In fact, many patients seeking hyperthermia in traditional hospitals end up getting more radiation and chemotherapy than they expected.

Q: What is Pulse Modulated Microwave Hyperthermia?

A: This is a special technology researched and developed by the combined efforts of Drs. Alsleben and Donsbach. It is a special modification of the generators producing the microwave energy and the computer software programs that control its delivery to the tumor. We intend to maintain an exclusivity on this technology until it can evolve to its highest perfection rather than have what we believe will be the most effective form of high energy healing suppressed and ridiculed by those who didn't think of it first. Simply stated, it is a method of using a portion of the microwave energy to carry specific tumor regressive instructions to the DNA code of the cancer cells.

Q: Can hyperthermia be used to treat rectal-colon, vaginal, breast, lung and prostate cancers?

A: Of course. Our Pulse Modulated Microwave Hyperthermia unit can treat cancer anywhere in the body. Obviously, some tumor locations are easier and more effectively treated. For example, a skin tumor would be far easier to treat than a tumor deep in the liver. A breast tumor would be easier to treat than a brain tumor, but something can be done to any tumor, and remember, heat is not the only modality we use. Our wholistic approach is astonishingly effective without hyperthermia. Imagine what could happen if the microwave increased our effectiveness by 10% or 50% or 100%. We have special applicator antennae that are used to treat tumors in the rectal-colon and vagina. We even have a second totally separate unit to treat prostate and bladder problems.

Q: Can microwave hyperthermia be used to treat an enlarge prostate gland?

A: Absolutely! And very effectively? Our microwave unit, specifically designed to treat prostate enlargement, does so by placing a very small antenna applicator right next to the prostate. How effective is the therapy? The easiest way to answer that question is to tell you about a study performed at the Mayo Clinic and reported in May of 1992. Sixty patients with severe enlargement of their prostate glands, causing major obstruction to urine flow, were treated with one 40 minute treatment of microwave hyperthermia. 100% of the patients returned to normal in the weeks following the treatment. That's how effective the therapy is. In fact, it was that report that convinced us to make the major capital investment required to obtain the equipment for our patients.

26

Q: When should a person with prostate enlargement be treated with microwave hyperthermia?

A: As soon as possible! Dr. Donsbach and I have emphasized prevention rather than crisis medicine all during our careers. Any fool can diagnose a severely enlarged prostate when the urine flow stops, but it is very difficult to detect it prior to symptoms.

Here are some facts about prostate cancer:

86,000 new cases of prostate cancer per year.
25% of the new cases of prostate cancer will die.
Most common cancer in men = lung.
Second most common cancer in men = prostate.
Prostate cancer increasing in the last four years.
Current traditional therapies are now being questioned.
Incidence for black race is 50% higher than whites.
Starting at age 50, the incidence doubles with each
  additional 5 years.
There may be decades between the tumor becoming
  malignant and the appearance of clinical symptoms.
The younger the onset, the shorter the life.
The more sexual activity, the higher the cancer incidence.
The relationship between BPH and cancer is uncertain.
Pattern of development of prostate cancer is very
  unpredictable.
40% of patients presenting with symptoms have
  advanced disease.
45% of patients presenting with symptoms have
  metastases.
Only symptoms are urinary flow changes. This is a

late symptom because adenocarcinoma is in the periphery of the gland.

Symptoms of advanced disease: urinary hesitancy, frequency, nocturia, incomplete emptying or dysuria. These symptoms are reported in only 60% of the cases. The first symptoms may be those of metastases to bone, etc.

The acknowledged most accurate diagnostic procedure for prostatic cancer is digital palpation. This means that the cancer is very likely metastatic long before it is large enough to palpate.

Any area of firmness, asymmetry or induration should be considered suspicious for carcinoma.

50% of prostatic nodules are malignant.

Stages of prostate cancer:

Stage A - no symptoms, no clinical findings, negative lab, carcinoma

Stage B - no symptoms, nodule, negative lab, carcinoma

Stage C - no symptoms or early urinary, extensive induration, might be urethral obstruction, might be acid phosphatase, carcinoma

Stage D - bone pain, urinary symptoms, variable induration, metastases, maybe acid phosphatase, maybe alkaline phosphatase

Five year survival of untreated case is 25%

Lymph node metastases:

22% for Stage A

54% for Stage B

77% for Stage C

Metastases by lymph and blood to bone, lung, liver and adrenal.

Now consider this awesome thought. Cancer in the prostate gland can become malignant and spread to other areas while it is still microscopic in size without presenting any symptoms at all. This tells us that males over the age of 40 should seriously consider preventive treatment for cancer of the prostate with the use of microwave hyperthermia. We believe that it is entirely possible for prostate cancer to metastasize to bone or lung before it is detectable in the prostate.

Our response in all forms of cancer have increased dramatically since the hyperthermia equipment was installed. We are pleased to offer this excellent therapy along with all the other therapies we use at our facilities.

TOTAL THYMUS EXTRACT THERAPY

The thymus gland is the headquarters of the immune system. It is the staging area for the maturation of T-lymphocytes, one of your principal cancer cell fighters. Computer projections indicate that the thymus gland may produce as many as 26 hormonal messengers related to defense, repair and rejuvenation. If the thymus gland is functioning properly, it is unlikely that disease processes would exist. Cancer therapy should include thymus therapy and thymus gland restoration.

HYDRAZINE SULFATE

One of the greatest discoveries of our time was the work of Dr. Otto Warburg who was awarded the Nobel Prize for his discovery that the major difference between normal cells and cancer cells was the fact that the energy production of one required oxygen and the other did not. Quite obviously, the normal cell requires oxygen to produce energy. The cancer cell utilizes a different methodology which we shall discuss as basically as possible.

Both the normal cell and the cancer cell utilize glucose as the raw material which is necessary for energy production, but there the similarity ceases. While the normal cell combines oxygen with glucose and yields 30 energy units for each molecule of glucose, the breakdown of glucose without oxygen in the cancer cell yields only 2 energy units per molecule of glucose. The anaerobic (without oxygen) breakdown also yields a high quantity of lactic acid which the liver and, to some extent, the kidney can convert into glucose again.

But here is where the significant and interesting weakness of the cancer cell becomes apparent. Since the yield of energy from glucose is so low in the cancer cell, it follows that the cancer cell must have an enormous appetite for glucose. This stimulates the liver and kidneys to produce more glucose from the lactic acid waste of cancer metabolism. The production of one molecule of glucose only furnishes 2 energy units for the cancer cell. Thus, the more cancer cells there are, the more the energy loss is to the normal cells of the body.

This inefficient conversion creates the cachetic state so often seen in cancer and from which more patients die than from the cancer itself. Properly defined, the cachetic state is one in which the normal cells of the body begin to waste away while the cancer cells flourish.

LET'S STARVE THE CANCER CELL

Since normal cells easily get their energy production from the glucose produced by the food we eat and are very efficient at it (15 times more efficient than a cancer cell) and the cancer cell is constantly calling upon the liver to create more glucose for its consumption, it should stand to reason that one could put the cancer cell at a significant disadvantage if one would inhibit the production of glucose from lactic acid in the liver.

This is exactly what hydrazine sulfate does and, although this will affect the normal cells to some degree, the cancer cell is so much more vulnerable that the use of hydrazine sulfate has been determined to be a safe and effective means of controlling the spread of cancer and has even reversed rather large tumor masses in many instances.

The simplicity of hydrazine sulfate is in its inhibitory effect on the enzyme which makes it possible to convert lactic acid into glucose. One might draw a parallel between the missing enzyme in the human liver which prevents us from making Vitamin C but, because it is present in animals, allows the manufacture of Vitamin C from glucose. In the presence of hydrazine sulfate, phosphoenolpyruvate carboxykinase (the enzyme necessary to convert lactic acid into glucose) is activated and glucose cannot be formed from lactic acid.

NOTICEABLE EFFECTS

Some of the most noticeable effects from the use of hydrazine sulfate are:

increased appetite   feeling of well being
mood elevation   decrease in tumor size
increase in strength   reduction in pain
decrease in lymph engorgement

Because of this extensive research, I have made the decision to use hydrazine sulfate in all cancer cases under therapy at the hospital.

HIDDEN CANCER CELLS

Cancer cells have the capacity to deploy decoys and masking chemicals that interfere with the immune system's efforts to find and attack them. Many of these molecules can be filtered from the blood, thereby enabling the immune system components to penetrate the cancer cells' "defense shields."

CESIUM CHLORIDE

The basic mechanism of cancer was outlined by Nobel Laureate Otto Warburg, who indicated that if a normal cell is disturbed by either radiation or a carcinogen, a free-radical induced change takes place in the cell. This change prevents oxygen from entering the cell, but glucose enters freely. Since glucose requires oxygen to produce energy, the glucose cannot produce energy in the cancer cell efficiently and is primarily metabolized into lactic acid.

This lactic acid induces an acid medium in the cell which now causes changes in the DNA of the cell and allows uninhibited reproduction. In addition, toxic enzymes are produced which accelerate the spreading or metastases of tumor cells. With this in mind, it is easy to see why surgery, radiation and chemotherapy are grossly ineffective in the treatment of this disease.

Many researchers have attempted to alter this acid proclivity of the cancer cell but, most substances used produced an alkalinity that was detrimental to the healthy cells and could not be used in high doses to control the cancer cell. Dr. Keith Brewer proposed that the use of cesium or rubidium would alter the pH of the cell without being toxic to normal cells and called his theory, "High pH Therapy for Cancer."

By giving cesium to cancer patients, the cesium specifically enters the cancer cell and makes the inside of the cell alkaline. Since all cancer cells are acid and raising the pH makes it increasingly difficult to continue reproduction, the therapy quickly slows down the growth. It is concluded that when the pH of the cell becomes 7.6, every cancer cell growth pattern is stopped and at a pH of 8 to 8.5, the life cycle of the cancer cell is limited to only a few hours.

When we became aware of this, we immediately began

to research data which substantiated the theory. The following is a partial list of the documentation.

a. Texas Tech University found that the use of cesium is most effective in the suppression and regression of sarcoma.

b. Hans Neiper, M.D., from Germany, is highly impressed with the use of cesium and says it is the treatment of choice in any kind of tumor, particularly bronchogenic carcinoma with bone metastasis.

c. American University of Washington D.C. indicated that tumors treated with cesium weighed only 9% as much as control tumors in animals not treated with cesium.

d. A 97% suppression of colon cancer was achieved by the use of cesium by the University of Wisconsin.

e. H.E. Sartori, M.D. found evidence of some shrinkage in tumor size in all cases in a study of 65 human patients with cancer. He also reported relief from pain in many instances.

Such evidence should not be overlooked and I am impressed enough to offer this therapy to all our cancer patients since there are practically no side effects and no cross purpose with any of the other wholistic remedies which we utilize.

SYNERGISTIC CANCER THERAPY

A remarkable discovery has been made. Some cancer effective medications and nutrients work better when given in combinations. Sometimes the combined beneficial effect is three or four times greater than when the substances are given singly. The is called synergism. Medical journal articles document the effects of synergism as follows:

Reduces malignant cell reproduction
Increases natural cancer killer cell activity
Stimulates the immune system
Increases defense of normal cells against cancer
Increases anti-tumor efficiency of chemotherapy
Activates white cell macrophages
Increases natural immunity
Direct anti-cancer effect
Improves quality of life
Induces long-term remission
Improves T-Helper cell responses
Enhances T cell growth factor
Selectively inhibits suppressor T cell function
Increases survival
Slows tumor growth
Direct tumorcidal effect
Arrests cancer cell growth
Helps to repair excessive damage from radiation and chemotherapy

Synergistic therapy is used at Hospital Santa Monica.

THERAPIES USED AT
HOSPITAL SANTA MONICA
HAVE BEEN PUBLISHED!

Cancer Treatment Reports
Seminars in Oncology
FDA Drug Bulletin
Center for Drugs and Biologics, Food & Drug Admin.
Journal of the American Medical Association
Physician's Desk Reference
British Journal of Cancer
Immunobiology
Cancer, Immunology, Immunotherapy
Chemotherapy
Cancer
International Colloquium on Bacteria & Cancer
Cancer Research Institute
New England Journal of Medicine
Nordic Medical Publications, Sweden
International Journal of Cancer
Acta Radio-Oncology
European Journal of Haematology
Journal of Cancer Research & Clinical Oncology
Diagnostic Immunology
Investigation of New Drugs
Journal of Biological Response Modifiers
Annals of Internal Medicine
International Journal of Radiation & Oncologic
Biologic Journal of Immuno-Pharmacology
Clinical Experimental Metastasis
Archives of Otolaryngologic Head & Neck Surgery
Journal of Laboratory & Clinical Medicine

LAETRILE

This substance probably epitomizes alternative cancer therapy more than any other in the minds of most citizens. Although it is my opinion that it has had its peak and there are now many other approaches of equal or superior value, there can be no doubt that the use of laetrile is a standard for most alternative clinics.

Laetrile was developed by Ernst Krebs, Jr., Ph.D. His discovery was centered around John Beard's theory that cancer grows from misplaced trophoblast cells. Trophoblasts are rapidly multiplying cells existing in a pregnant human uterus during the first weeks after conception.

These trophoblasts are usually killed off by chymotrypsin, a pancreatic enzyme, but any cells escaping this fate will lodge in the developing embryo. They may live for decades in almost any part of the body, ready to develop into cancer whenever the pancreas begins to fail. This is probably the best theory to explain the appearance of cancer in a non-drinking, non-smoking, health food enthusiast who exercises every day. Laetrile does the work of chymotrypsin by combining with betaglucuronidase, an enzyme that destroys excess estrogen produced by all cancer cells. Several new chemicals are formed, one of which is hydrocyanic acid, containing the poison cyanide. Normal cells have the ability to produce another enzyme, rhodanase, which deactivates small amounts of cyanide, but cancer cells are unable to produce rhodanase. In this way, hydrocyanic acid from laetrile kills the cancer cells, not normal cells, leaving behind no harmful side effects.

Laetrile is taken either as a preventive or as part of a full metabolic treatment against cancer. This ingredient is found in over 1,200 different plants, particularly in the seeds of common fruits, such as apricots, peaches, plums and apples. It is available in both injectable and tablet forms and can be purchased for about $10 per vial (3 grams) or $85 per 100 - 500 milligram tablets.

Although opponents are always shrieking about the toxicity of the cyanide released, the clinical facts indicate that toxicity in the usual doses of 3 to 6 grams per day is non-existent.

INTERFERON

When a cell is infected with a virus, it manufactures and secretes chemical messengers that signal neighboring cells as to how to defend themselves. These are called interferons. It is now known that interferons can inhibit growth of cancer cells, if the correct dosage is used. Interferons stimulate T-lymphocytes. The action of interferon is increased when combined with butyrate and urea compounds.

GERMANIUM

When I think of germanium, I subconsciously think of Japanese Shitake Mushrooms, ginseng, garlic and other folk remedies which have survived the test of time and thus impress me with the fact that something beneficial is going on or such use would have been designated to the scrap heap long ago. All of these plants are rich in germanium. Whether germanium is the only active ingredient in these plants is certainly debatable, but the fact remains that these are healing plants and germanium alone has proved to be a highly successful adjunct in the treatment of cancer.

Otto Warburg, Nobel Laureate, said "Cancer, above all other disease, has countless secondary causes. But there is only one prime cause. Summarized in a few words, THE PRIME CAUSE OF CANCER IS THE REPLACEMENT OF THE NORMAL OXYGEN RESPIRATION OF BODY CELLS BY ANAEROBIC (without oxygen) CELL RESPIRATION." Dr. Szent Gyorgyi also felt that cancer originated from an insufficient oxygen supply.

It must, therefore, follow that a substance which can increase the amount of oxygen in the tissue will also reduce the chance of cancer beginning. Since anaerobic cells cannot live in a high-oxygen environment, the use of a substance which enhances oxygen could also be a factor in curing the problem. Germanium is an oxygen enhancer and we give it to every patient we work with. All of the staff doctors are also convinced that results have increased since we began using germanium.

There is an extensive research which indicates that another mode of action of germanium lies in its ability to stimulate the body's own natural defense system. Reported in the *Journal of Interferon Research #4*, 1984: "Organic germanium treated test animals show an inhibitory effect against certain tumors in such a way that would suggest that the effect is the result of increased macrophage activity."

The *Tohoku Journal of Experimental Medicine* said "The anti-tumor action of organic germanium appears to be related to its interferon-inducing activity."

At a cost of $25 per 10 cc vial, this medicine is an attractive way to prevent and/or treat cancer. 150 mg oral tablets are about $1.50 each with three or more being the daily dosage.

DMSO
(DiMethyl Sulfoxide)

DMSO is possibly the best solvent in the world. But of more interest to our readers, it has an almost unbelievable variety of applications of pain relief in a hundred diseases and conditions. It has been used safely and successfully by millions of people around the world to control inflammation and swelling, reduce pain, slow the growth of bacteria, viruses and fungi, relieve burns sprains, strains and arthritis. It has relieved the symptoms of shingles and other forms of herpes, tuberculosis, sinusitis and **even** cancer.

At Hospital Santa Monica, we use DMSO in our "basic" infusion, which consists of hydrogen peroxide and DMSO. Every patient gets this because I have found that DMSO helps mitigate the irritation some feel with the hydrogen peroxide, as well as providing the benefits that DMSO has all by itself.

At New York's Mt. Sinai Hospital, it was discovered that when DMSO was injected into leukemic mice, the leukemic cancer cells began to perform as normal cells. In this form of cancer, the body is inundated with immature white cells which do not mature. More and more are formed because the body is desperate to have a normal amount of defense. It appears that, in some way, DMSO caused the immature cells to "grow up" and become functional.

It is my personal opinion that DMSO assists all the other substances I use in the treatment of cancer, as well as having specific actions of its own. The Food and Drug Administration has succeeded in keeping this beneficial medication from the general public. There are "solvent" grade products available which, in general, are acceptable but carry the risk of being contaminated and carrying such contamination into the body because of the excellent solvent properties of this substance. Hopefully we will soon see medical-grade product available. Any DMSO side effects that you may have heard about are, in my opinion, not valid. Extensive research has authenticated its safety in human use.

WHAT IS ONCOTOX?

OncoTox contains an ortho-para-toluene-sul-fonamide compound with the organic formula $C_9H_{13}O_2NS$. **OncoTox** is non-toxic at therapeutic doses and has specific and measurable cancer cell killing and growth inhibitor effects via both the IM and oral routes. At the Mallory Institute of Pathology, Boston School of Medicine, **OncoTox** has been shown to enhance both B and T cell responses to mitogens and enhance natural killer cell activity.

In controlled studies, **Onco Tox** clearly demonstrated inhibition of tumor growth and mitosis in only four days. Thus, **OncoTox** has a specific "killer" effect on cancer cells and inhibits their reproduction, but doesn't not have any such effect on normal cells.

CLODRONATE

After several frustrating years of trying, I was able to procure a product which is a light shinning in the dark for the bone cancer patient. Bone cancer is usually a metastatic transplant of a primary breast or prostate cancer. It is a known fact by oncologists that either one of these cancers will result in bone metastasis in 80% of the cases they see.

Until clodronate was discovered, there was little that

could be done, since bone cancer is very resistant to any form of chemotherapy or even radiation, although this will slow down the growth temporarily. In this form of cancer, the bone is actually thinned, with an excess amount of calcium being found in the blood.

The pain that bone cancer patients eventually experience is one of the most resistant pains known. Even the high doses of morphine soon become impotent against this excruciating pain. Although I have not always found it to work this rapidly, most bone cancer patients are pain tolerant within 36 to 48 hours of administering clodronate.

A fairly new medicine, clodronate is essentially side effect free and extremely effective in altering the outflow of calcium that occurs from the bone. Thus, it prevents further metastasis, which is the dream of everyone who treats bone cancer. This cancer has a nasty habit of jumping from the spine to the ribs to the skull to the pelvis, etc. There is adequate evidence to understand how these "seed" cells travel in the bone, since there are microcapillaries in the bone marrow that literally have gaps in them that could be entry points for cancer cells.

Clodronate thus offers two great advances in the treatment of bone cancer - it reduces pain and prevents the condition from spreading. There is inadequate evidence that it actually cures bone cancer, but remission and containment are a satisfactory substitute. It must be used continuously, but the dosages can be gradually reduced. It is quite expensive, being in the $400 per month range. The patient needs to make the decision to use it since it is the only medicine we know of that is effective.

A COMMON QUESTION

"When is it too late to come to Hospital Santa Monica?

Answer: I have no way of knowing. Experience has taught me that sometimes the most hopeless appearing cases do far better than a patient who exhibits far less serious effects. If everyone else has given up and you still want to try to "beat" it, who has the right to judge or the knowledge to predict the outcome. Miracles at Hospital Santa Monica are all too common to say it won't happen to you.

HYDROGEN PEROXIDE

This may well be the most difficult of all the therapies to write about since we do not wish to lead anyone astray or make claims which cannot be sustained. Our hospital does not have the facilities or the resources to do pure research. Therefore, what we write about is clinical observation which is often referred to as "anecdotal" evidence in the realm of "science." We have often pondered why it is that if a response is repeatable enough times to be predictable, it is still considered "anecdotal" until the man of "science" has put his blessing upon it. We believe this is purely a control mechanism on the part of those who control medicine.

On the other hand, we do have considerable printed evidence from sacrosanct medical journals to justify the stand we take on this subject. A study by Sasake, Wakutani, Oda and Yamasaki from the Tottori University School of Medicine, explores the known fact that the therapeutic effect of radiation is enhanced by increasing the oxygen tension in the cell. Ordinary methods of increasing oxygen were considered faulty so they devised an experiment where hydrogen peroxide was infused prior to radiation therapy and later prior to the use of chemotherapy.

Since the purpose of the infusion was to increase the oxygen tension in the cancer cell, the infusions were carried out for 10 consecutive days. Of 15 cases of maxillary cancer, 8 showed almost complete disappearance of the tumor, 6 demonstrated a partial reduction and only 1 had little change. Most of the cases which showed significant response to the infusion began to show rapid fusion and sloughing of the tumor in the cavity 3-4 days after the start of the infusion. In these cases, the tumor turned into a state similar to pasty bean-curd, making it impossible to recognize the original state of the tumor. Those cases which showed partial reduction of tumor mostly developed necrosis from either outside or the front part of the cavity and gradually tended to be reduced and circumscribed.

In addition, 3 cases complaining of stubborn trigeminal neuralgia before the start of the treatment showed disappearance of pain after 3-4 days. The Japanese researchers concluded, "Since these shockingly good results have given us confidence, we have decided to continue clinical studies on the method."

It was this type of report, echoed by others, which gave me the confidence to use hydrogen peroxide as an infusion. When I announced it, there was an immediate barrage of cautionary advise from friends and colleagues who warned me of the dangers of a gas bubble (emboli) resulting from the hydrogen peroxide. This is a logical assumption, particularly since the oxidation effect of hydrogen peroxide does produce bubbles. I am happy to report that literature searches do not reveal this as a problem and practical experience in over ten thousand infusions performed at Hospital Santa Monica has resulted in not one single case.

In pioneering this technique on a broad scale, I became

46

so confident and impressed with the results of the infusion of hydrogen peroxide that I began using it in every conceivable form of disease known to man with some startlingly (good) results.

Let me share with you an "anecdote."

Mrs. A. H. was admitted to Hospital Santa Monica with the words of her doctors ringing in her ears, "You just have a very short few weeks of life, prepare yourself and your family. There is nothing more that medicine can do for you." She had cancer of the lung with metastasis to several other areas. For the first 10 days, it seemed as if the prophesy would come true. We shared with her husband that she did indeed seem to be deteriorating and we gave a dim prognosis. By the end of the 3rd week, she had obtained a complete turn around and was doing so well that her husband left her side and went back to work, confident that his wife would live. By the end of the 4th week, this lady was on the tennis court for 45 minutes.

Her remarkable recovery may sound miraculous, it is not intended to be, but it is an often repeated happenstance at the Hospital. We have to give much credit to hydrogen peroxide, even though we use many other remedies, as outlined in this book.

In summary of hydrogen peroxide, we have to make certain statements.

1. Cancer cells are less virulent and may even be

destroyed by the presence of a high oxygen environment.

2. Hydrogen peroxide given by infusion and orally has the ability to increase the oxygen content of the blood stream which will increase the oxygen environment of the cancer cell.

3. Clinical evidence has overwhelmingly convinced me that the use of hydrogen peroxide is a valuable adjunct in the treatment of cancer.

The infusion we use must be carefully prepared or there will be pain and destruction of red blood cells. I caution anyone to learn the protocol before attempting to use this approach. Oral administration is a problem only in that the taste of hydrogen peroxide is awful. Many people get very nauseated and even vomit. Fortunately, there is a product on the market which overcomes these side effects. For further information on this subject, see the book entitled O_2 O_2 O_2.

CO Q-10

CoEnzyme Q-10 is not a newcomer to the cancer field - it has been used with toxic chemotherapy to help mitigate its side effects. There is a very critical dosage level for chemotherapy in that the dosage necessary to kill a cancer cell will often kill healthy cells as well. A comparatively effective anti-cancer drug is Adriamycin, but this drug is very difficult to administer because many of the patients who had it administered end up with serious heart ailments. Researchers found that

Adriamycin depleted the Co Q-10 in the heart muscle and when Co Q-10 was administered in conjunction with the drug, heart damage did not occur.

Work at the New England Institute measured the clearance of foreign matter from the blood circulation with and without Co Q-10 supplementation. Such foreign material was removed twice as fast in Co Q-10 treated individuals as compared to those who did not take the substance. Cancer patients are particularly vulnerable to accumulation of toxins and if Co Q-10 helps to remove them twice as fast, I'm all for it.

In a separate study, Co Q-10 treated animals developed tumors at a 31% slower rate than non-treated animals. This immune stimulation has been documented to produce a two-fold increase in the phagocytic rate and significantly increased the antibody levels. Mice inoculated with cancer and then treated with Co Q-10 or without it were monitored for life span. The Co Q-10 mice lived for 300 plus days, the untreated mice lived a maximum of 132 days.

To my knowledge, nobody is touting Co Q-10 as having anti-cancer activity per se, but the demonstrated enhancement of all the body functions that are involved in cancer control is certainly reason enough to utilize it. Most studies indicate that the effective dose is between 60 and 100 mg daily, with larger dosages not achieving any greater results. Because it is quite expensive, many formulae offer only low dosages, but higher potencies are available.

FLUTAMIDE

One of the most popular treatments for prostate cancer has been orchiectomy or removal of the testes. Some doctors prefer flooding the male body with high doses of estrogen to shut down the testes. All of this is based upon the assumption that the testosterone produced by the testes stimulate the growth of cancer, much as estrogen is believed to stimulate breast and uterine cancer.

Neither procedure is particularly welcome to the male. Surgical castration has a severe psychological effect on some; estrogen produces fluid retention, heart disease, thromboembolism and breast enlargement. It has been proposed that treatment with a leutinizing hormone releasing hormone (LHRH) would accomplish the same as either the surgery or the female hormone treatment without the side effects. Several hospitals have begun such use and report excellent blocking of the androgenic hormones from the testes.

The sad truth of the matter is that none of the above treatments are more than band-aids after about 6 months when androgenic hormone production by the adrenals begins to take over. According to Geller, Natchtsheim, Albert and Laza (Journal of Urology: 132-1984) approximately 50% of male hormone is produced by the adrenals. Furthermore, it is believed that upon either surgical or chemical castration, there is an upsurge of androgen production by the adrenals.

Dr. LaBrie initiated the use of Flutamide in the treatment of prostatic cancer and its metastatic after effects with some extremely dramatic results:

1. Signs and symptoms of cancer disappeared in all of 87 previously untreated patients in a test group.

2. 25% of the patients showed a complete disappearance of bone cancer.

3. 55% of the patients demonstrated at least 50% reduction in bone metastasis.

A 2 year study of these same patients showed an 81% remission rate as compared to 0% remission usually seen in patients treated in the orthodox fashion. Prostatic acid phosphatase levels are considered an excellent method of charting the progress of prostatic cancer. Within 5 days of initiating LHRH and Flutamide therapy, levels of this marker begin to decrease by as much as 50% and in 90% of the cases, this level will be normal within 2 months.

Although this is a very strong statement to make, it is my opinion that even advanced metastatic prostate cancer can now be put into remission using not only the 2 substances mentioned here, but also hydrogen peroxide infusion and Clodronate to close off the routes of this cancer.

There are exceptions, of course, and these will always be in the patients who have been treated with estrogens only for a period of time. The cancer cells transform into nonandrogenic dependent and the LHRH and Flutamide therapy is no longer beneficial. This does not mean that all the other methods discussed in this book would not be successful. It does mean the cancer would not react to LHRH or Flutamide.

This is the main reason we use so many different treatment avenues with every cancer patient. If one cannot work, another may well be able to fill the gap.

Flutamide is expensive, over $200 per month on a maintenance basis, but well worth it to keep prostate cancer at bay.

LIVE CELL THERAPY

There are many misconceptions about this therapy. Certain companies who sell, or the person promoting it, become intent on selling the "sizzle" rather than the steak.

Deep within every cell lies the DNA or "code of life." The exact structure of the cell involved is imprinted in the DNA. Upon the death of a cell, the DNA supervises the creation of an exact replica. Thus, a dying liver cell brings forth a vibrant new liver cell. Remember that a cancer cell is a normal cell which has had its DNA invaded, causing genetic changes, the most significant of which is the loss of growth control.

It is further believed that a number of circumstances such as drug abuse, alcohol, malnutrition, etc., could cause a sluggishness of the DNA. When this occurs, certain cells will not replace themselves and premature aging and dysfunction occur.

The use of extracted DNA from animal organs began many years ago and has progressively become more refined and effective. Unborn animals are used because their immune system has not had a chance to develop antibodies against all manner of possible dangers; so these extracts do not become antigens to incite an allergic response.

The premise is simple. The extracted DNA of liver, pancreas, thymus, adrenal, spleen or whatever organ, is injected as a natural stimulant into the individual's own DNA. We use it as a general stimulant (13 organ and gland extracts are used) to energize a slowed down and overworked body. Our patients need all the help they can get to overcome serious illness.

THYMUS GLAND

The headquarters of the immune system is the thymus gland, located beneath the breast bone in humans. The thymus gland may secrete as many as 26 hormones. Among those that have been isolated are hormones that control the growth of cells, levels of blood sugar and functions of white blood cells, especially the T-lymphocytes and natural killer cells. The thymus gland produces biochemical messengers that instruct lymphocytes and other white blood cells to attack cancer cells, destroy the body's enemies and effect repairs.

Among the messengers are natural interferon and interleukin compounds.

THYMUS ACTIVATION THERAPY

Thymus Activation Therapy, originally developed in Sweden more than 40 years ago, has been given to hundreds of thousands of patients with excellent results. In 1976, the first, and perhaps only, physician outside of Europe to be commissioned to deliver the therapy was H. Rudolph Alsleben, M.D. During the last 15 years, Dr. Alsleben has discovered numerous ways to improve its effectiveness. His joining the staff of Hospital Santa Monica has added many valuable years of experience to the care of our patients.

VITAMIN A & BETA-CAROTENE

Nutritionists have for years lauded the properties of Vitamin A and have been just as vigorously opposed by the "chosen guardians" of your health who have claimed that this nutrient is injurious to your health in any dosage except very minimal RDA (Recommended Daily Allowance). Even though a recent study has indicated at least 1/3 of all Americans are not getting the RDA of Vitamin A in their daily diet, regular press releases warn against using too much Vitamin A.

University studies have indicated that large amounts (600,000 IU daily) were not toxic when taken with Vitamin E, but such information is conveniently ignored. They have advocated increasing those foods in your diet which contain a precursor to Vitamin A (beta-carotene) because of overwhelming evidence that this substance (which changes to Vitamin A in the body) does indeed neutralize the changes in pre-cancerous tissue and revert such tissue back to normal.

Vitamin A is absolutely essential for the production of natural antibodies against cancer cells by the thymus. We use large amounts of both Vitamin A and beta-carotene at Hospital Santa Monica. There have never been any side effects noted and we have observed some fantastic results in rare cancer such as mycosis fungoides.

IMMUNE STIMULATION

The immune system in the body is both our watchdog and police system to control unwanted actions. We sincerely believe that if a person has a strong immune system, cancer has much less chance of obtaining a stranglehold on the body. It is my opinion that each and every one of us fight cancer cells every day. Based on this belief, I do not tell our patients that we "cure" cancer. I have seen so many disappointed patients who have been told by a surgeon, "We got it all." Our intent is to make the body so strong that cancer cells cannot survive and multiply without control as they used to do.

Since the thymus is the seat of the immune system, we pay a lot of attention to this gland, using various extracts, concentrated nutrients such as pantothenic acid, Vitamin A and other products to enhance its function.

Other glands and organs such as the spleen, the lymphatic circulation and bone marrow are similarly supported. We are constantly using products such as Interferon, Isoprinosine, BCG, Gamma Globulin and any other substance which has been proved to support and activate the immune system.

BIO-MAGNETIC & MICRO-FREQUENCIES

Some alternative practitioners have made the statement that many humans would be better off seeing their veterinarian than their medical doctor. This may be slightly tongue-in-check, but it is true that new advances are often tested through the animal kingdom before human testing is done. The above therapies are widespread in animal therapy in the United States and are quite widespread among the human population in Europe, often by alternative practitioners.

Much evidence exists that these energy waves assist healing and, in a beneficial way, stimulate energy forces in the body. Such stimulation in cases of stubborn fractures which will not heal for many months has convinced even the most skeptical.

Certain fields of thought hold that micro-frequencies have the ability to destroy abnormal cells and harmful organisms, depending upon the frequency used. Such reasoning has been with us for some time and the work of modern scientists are authenticating it. Since none of this conflicts with any other therapy and we have seen apparent miracles from its use, it is a constant in our program.

OTHER THERAPIES

If a therapy is brought to our attention and fulfills the requirements that it will not interfere with our known therapies and is relatively non-toxic, we begin to add such to selected patients to see if they do better with the substance than without it. The following are some therapies that have passed our test and are quite regularly used where indicated.

Carbatine - This therapy was developed by a physician in Greece, Dr. Demopoulas. It is based upon the healing effect of urine on certain conditions. Liver and bone cancers respond very well to the addition Carbatine to the treatment protocols. Carbatine contains urea and creatine hydrate, both of which have been shown to have anti-cancer properties. Both are remarkably non-toxic. A profound study was performed at the University of Illinois Medical Center.:

TUMOR MATRIX DESTRUCTION BY THE USE OF HYDROPHOBIC BREAKERS: A PRELIMINARY REPORT. Clinical Oncology 1977, 3, 319-320.

Malignant cells are known to consist of aggregations of deviant cells, the surfaces of which are rich in glycoprotein and other macromolecular surface-active agents. Through a combination of hydrophobic bonding at non-polar sites and water adsorption at hydrophilic sites, these surfactants form a highly structured matrix containing immobilized water and electrolytes in which cancer cells are embedded. This matrix is disrupted by the ingredients of Carbatine which leads to interference with metabolic exchanges and replication processes necessary for continued uncontrolled cellular growth. The effectiveness of urea against a variety of malignancies in both laboratory and clinical studies is extremely significant. The ability of this medicine to enter into anti-cancer synergisms with agents exerting similar matrix structure breaking effects is an additional significant property.

Shark Liver Extract - This substance was originally researched in Sweden as an answer to leukemia. Rather impressive evidence indicates it is effective in other cancers as well.

Shark Cartilage Extract - It came to the attention of researchers many years ago that sharks do not develop cancer. In searching for a reason, an enterprising young biochemist rationalized that a characteristic of the shark not shared by other fish is that the skeleton is made up only of cartilage, not bone.

Hard work and many disappointments led him to discover a factor in shark cartilage that inhibits the formation of new blood vessels. Since all cells require a plentiful blood supply, and tumor cells are no exception, the inhibition or stopping of such needed new blood vessels will effectively stop growth and allow other measures to be more effective in reducing the cancer.

More and more evidence documenting the success of this approach is surfacing every month.

Micro-Dose Chemotherapy - The concept of chemotherapy is quite logical - use a substance which will kill the cancer cell. The great drawback of this has been that in destroying the cancer cell, normal cells are also destroyed. Giving enough chemotherapy to kill the cancer cell and not kill the body has been the great challenge. The side effect for which this therapy is so well known for is the destruction of normal cells which occurs when the quantity necessary to kill the cancer cells is used. Small doses are not effective because they will not destroy enough cancer cells to make a difference.

However, using the therapies which have been outlined in this book, a micro-dosage has been found to be effective without the side effect of the larger dosages. Also, as we have pointed out, several of the approaches we use neutralize the side effects of chemotherapy.

It has been necessary, when we have a cancer that is spreading so rapidly that we are concerned we cannot stop it in time, to discuss with the patient the possibility of using micro-dosages of certain chemotherapeutic agents. This approach has been effective, as has micro-dosage radiation, where indicated. We feel it is our responsibility to use whatever method is best for the patient.

The Drops of Life - The sometimes heroic measures we use at Hospital Santa Monica would not be appropriate and certainly not necessary for the average individual. But, we treat terminal illness with the intent of restoring that body to normal social life. We are not interested in making the last few days of a person's life more comfortable. Our job is to restore normalcy to a chaotic and depressed body.

On the premise that we cannot rebuild cells of any kind, much less those of the immune system without amino acids, all of our infusions contain a concentrated free amino acid solution. This gives strength as well as building blocks for repair and rejuvenation. For certain seriously debilitated patients, we will use this amino acid infusion on a daily basis.

In addition to these amino acids, our infusion will contain B complex vitamins, Vitamin C, calcium, magnesium, potassium and a broad spectrum of trace mineral elements. Although we supplement freely in oral form, many are not able to swallow tablets or to assimilate them even though they can swallow.

We call this super mixture "The Drops of Life" because it is so loaded with the various nutrients necessary for life.

NUTRITION

There are few areas in the treatment of cancer that arouse more dogmatic opinions than the area of nutrition. To fast or not to fast, to eat meat of any kind or to be a true vegetarian, to avoid dairy products or enjoy them, to drink copious amounts of juice or to drink little if any, to eat fruits for breakfast or to eat or not eat protein of any kind, the list is endless.

Each opinion has its staunch advocates, some to the point of being absolute fanatics. Maybe we mellow a bit as we age or maybe experience teaches us a basic lesson - moderation in all things seems to win more than dogmatism.

Probably the most difficult question I have to answer is from the health enthusiast who says, "Doctor, I've never smoked or drank alcohol, I watch my diet consistently and I know a lot about nutritional supplements and have used them regularly - why do I have cancer?"

On the other side of the coin, we all know of those who have abused their bodies unmercifully with every imaginable negative and who don't have or get cancer.

This has to lead us to believe that we all have some potential cancer cells in our body. Many factors can activate such dormant cells, much as a virus like the chicken pox virus can hide in the nervous system for 60 to 70 years and then manifest itself as herpes zoster or shingles in later life. Certainly genetics has an influence, however, so does diet but, it is not the only factor.

Thus it has been my practice to give the cancer patient a broad range of foods which can be used if they so desire. There is no question that certain individuals tolerate certain foods much better than others. Nordic-Germanic ancestry usually gives one the constitution to use meats and dairy products well, but seems to create problems if soy in introduced in any quantity in the diet. There are others who feel sluggish and generally not well if they consume a considerable portion of meats or dairy products. We cannot impose vegetarianism on everyone, some just are not physiologically adapted to it.

So my moderate rules for good health include lots of "do's" and very few "don't's." In this way, if you follow my "do's," you won't have the room for the "don't's." Here they are:

1. If you are going to fast, do it very cautiously and not for over 3 days without **competent** supervision. A competent person is not one who routinely advocates long fasts. If you have cancer, you need food to build your immune system and give yourself the energy to feel good.

2. Eat 4 cupfuls of vegetables daily. There are no hard and fast rules as to which vegetables, but if you follow this, you will find that you will automatically choose a wider and wider variety.

3. Eat one serving of oatmeal daily. It is an excellent high fiber cereal with a special fiber which is a help in reducing the fats in the system.

4. Refrain from unsaturated oils and from margarine totally. These have been implicated in a higher incidence

of cancer in heavy users.

5. Reduce coffee intake to a maximum of 1 cup daily, do try to learn the herb tea habit.

6. The consumption of refined sugars is the worst food for a cancer victim there is. Use whole fruits instead. If you must "sin," set aside 1 day a week in which you consume the "don't" foods. You will soon find that they don't taste as good as you thought they would and since you know that you can have them, but just not now, the prohibition is not that difficult.

7. Try to eat your best meals early in the day and avoid heavy meals at night.

8. Do not combine fruits and fruit juices with concentrated proteins (meats, dairy products, eggs), this will produce gas and discomfort.

9. Be positive and happy when you eat, your digestion will be better.

10. Eat 5 servings of chicken, fish or turkey each week, more if you are comfortable with it, less if you are not. Eat eggs and dairy products in moderation, if desired.

Food is such an individual factor in one's life that we hesitate to create drastic changes. There are enough other factors that enter into recovery, one of the most important is relaxation and a lack of stress. Denial of a favorite food can be extremely stressful to some and hinder their recovery. Until someone can prove that the consumption of any particular food causes cancer, we will continue to take the moderate approach.

One procedure we really like to see is that of washing all fruits, vegetables, fish and meats in a 3% solution of hydrogen peroxide to remove as much contaminant as possible. Such a solution can be used for several batches of foods so it ends up being a relatively inexpensive way to purify your foods and even remove some pesticide residue if you must purchase commercial vegetables and fruits.

IN CONCLUSION

History has proven to me that what I write today could have been done better tomorrow because there is always something new which could alter that which you have written. Such thinking would result in zero publications, so I freely admit that by the time you read this, some research will have probably occurred that resulted in a "new" therapy for the cancer patient.

I can only assure you that if such comes about, I will assess it and make a decision as to whether it becomes part of the armamentarium of Hospital Santa Monica. Much of our new information comes from our patients, since they have the greatest incentive to learn all there is to know about cancer. If you know of something that you feel is really worthwhile, please share it with me.

But a word of caution - the cancer patients we see are

seriously and often terminally ill. Kitchen remedies just aren't enough at this stage. I am bombarded with claims about what probably are good herbs, algae, etc., but most of our patients have tried that route and found they needed something more. Not to say that something simple might not be the answer. Hydrogen peroxide is a good example of a simple substance with powerful abilities.

As more and more of our patients leave and go back home, more and more clinical testing of the alternative approach to cancer is being accomplished. If all of our patients die, then we should not continue our efforts. Our records indicate that a high percentage of those who leave here are alive years after they had their treatment. That in itself is a small miracle since they were usually terminal when they came.

But what really puts the icing on the wholistic cake is the doctor who asks with incredulity, "What have you been doing? Your cancer is almost gone!" and when told that alternative methodology was employed, dismisses the patient and says that they would not like to see them again. Instead of being interested in what brought about this miracle, they are so prejudiced that they are unwilling to even listen.

Some of our patients have put a letter to the editor of their local newspapers when this occurs. It just might help some other individual who has been told there is no hope.

THERE DEFINITELY IS HOPE!
BUT ONLY YOU
CAN INITIATE THE
HEALING EXPERIENCE!

— · — · — · —

IMMUNE-MODULATION THERAPY
BREAKTHROUGH IN CANCER THERAPY

Darkfield microscopy of fresh human blood by such scientific giants as Villique in France, von Brehmer in Germany, Fonte in Italy, Livingston and Alsleben in California, have repeatedly demonstrated luminous micro-organisms in the bloodstream of patients suffering from catastrophic diseases. These organisms have been isolated, identified and casually related to various collagen and tumorous diseases. Many of the previous observations have in reality been of the same organism only in different forms. Some of the more recent names given to the organism are Bacillus Endoparasiticus, the T-bacillus and possibly the Progenitoracae Cryptocides. The organism has been cultured from tissues and bodily fluids of all tumor-bearing hosts, both human and animal. The organism is pleomorphic, it is capable of assuming different shapes and forms, dependent upon the environment in which it lives, that environment being your body. The organism seems to be present in all people. In some people, the organism appears very scanty; only a few dancing white specks can be seen under the darkfield microscope. Yet in others, it is present in such abundance that the red blood cells themselves are jolted by their movement.

In 1934, Dr. von Brehmer isolated a specific organism from human blood which he called the SIPHONSPORA POLYMOR-PHA. He believed that this organism could very well be the basic cause of all illness. In later years of research, it was found that if the acid pH level of the blood became more alkaline, i.e., from 7.35 to 7.45, the organism became identifiable with tumor growth. Just think of how incredible this statement is! A change of just 1/10th of a point toward alkalinity and cancer begins? He was able to culture the organism from many human tumors as well as the blood of the person with the tumors. The more that von Brehmer searched, the more places within the body the organism could be found. The organism is highly pleomorphic and capable of changing into mycelia fungal forms, sporangia and spore forms.

Dr. Alsleben and I have researched these organism for many years using special darkfield microscopic techniques and time-lapse motion picture photography that revealed where they come from, where they go and what they do in the meantime. We observed a family of nearly submicroscopic life forms in the blood of cancer victims that are definitely associated with many degenerative diseases, especially cancer. These organisms exist in all people all the time, but like tax collectors, they only gather in force when they need energy, which they cannot make themselves. If your internal biochemical environment supports their growth, they will grow; at the expense of your life.

There are two very devastating features about these miniature life forms. Imagine trillions of microscopic cannibals munching away at your cells and precious bodily fluids, robbing you of your life energies and giving you waste products in return. And the waste products themselves are vicious little chemicals that weaken cell membranes everywhere to the point where they leak away their vital nutrients. We know that these Kleptic ™ microbes rob energy from our cells, that they are toxic to every cell and that Kleptic microbes are capable of altering the DNA instructions within our tissue cells. We know that if they colonize in joint membranes, the result will be arthritis. If they attack the skin, the result is psoriasis. If they set up housekeeping in an organ, the result will be cancer.

Many courageous investigators have attempted to create vaccines to aid the defenses of the body against this internal corrosion without complete success. Now in our time, a step closer to the ultimate has been achieved. Through the auspices of the AL-DON MEDICAL RESEARCH INSTITUTE, we have achieved the following breakthroughs in immune modulator blueprints. We can now provide:

1. A general <u>cancer</u> immune modulator;

2. A specific <u>rheumatoid arthritis</u> immune modulator;

3. A specific <u>psoriasis</u> immune modulator;

4. An <u>autogenous vaccine</u> for the precursor of the deadly Progenitor Cryptocides cancer-related microbe identified by Livingston; and

5. A <u>purified antigen</u> for cancer.

Call for more information - 619-475-2874

SKIN CANCER

We have gone into great detail on the various aspects of cancer of and in the body. Another form of cancer which is on a rather spectacular increase in number is skin cancer. Some blame the depletion of the ozone layer, but we find that rather doubtful in light of the facts. There is very little doubt, however, that protracted exposure to the sun will produce a greater incidence of cancer as compared to the individual who stays in the shade.

There are three basic skin cancers:

1. **Squamous cell carcinoma** - This cancer is among the most common and the easiest to treat, as we shall see. It primarily originates from the outer cells of the epithelium.

2. **Basal cell carcinoma** - As the name suggests, this skin cancer comes from the deeper layers of the epidermis and is a little more difficult to treat.

3. **Melanoma** - A skin tumor of high malignancy that starts in a black mole and metastasizes rapidly and widely. One of the most feared of all cancers.

These cancers are most often seen after the age of 40 years and seem to increase with the years from there. The most common form of therapy is to surgically remove or burn them. All too often this is very temporary at best and the recurrence rate is very high. As noted before, melanoma is extraordinarily aggressive and, for many, the diagnosis of melanoma is the beginning of the end. **But there is another way!**

ESCHAROTICS

Escharotics belong to a group of compounds that are capable of producing a scab when applied to the skin. More specifically, when an escharotic is applied to visible cancer areas, the following sequence of events will occur.

First, there will be mass destruction of the cancer cells but not the normal cells.

Second, you will have pus formation with a scab forming over the area.

Third, there will be a sloughing off of the scab, leaving a

non-cancerous "pit" or cavity.

Fourth, all of this will heal over and leave a slightly de-pigmented area with a slight scar.

This entire procedure will take from 5 to 15 days on the average. The absolute most remarkable fact about this treatment is (to our knowledge) there has never been a single secondary infection from using the product which we use. There are several formulas on the market, some dating back almost 100 years with a basis of Indian folk lore.

All of them seem to work to some degree. The product we are familiar with is unique in that you only need to apply it once and sit back and wait for the 4 steps above to be completed. Almost all the other formulations must be applied several times and often 2 different salves are used.

The properties represented by these products are derived primarily from the following herbs: sanguinaria (bloodroot), bittersweet, ginger root, galangal, creosote bush and even capsicum. The more modern formulas contain zinc chloride as an anti-microbial, this makes sense. Inactive ingredients were only limited by the ingenuity of the formulator and ranged widely: kerosene, glycerine, lard, metallic cobalt, olive oil and water.

An amazing phenomenon is evident when one uses these formulations. If you have a suspicious skin growths, you can apply the escharotic ointment once and observe for a period of several days. In an "eschar" (pus which scabs over) forms, it is a cancer; if it doesn't, the growth is benign. Some doctors use this method to diagnose suspicious growths.

Although the escharotic ointment is capable of removing larger tumors from beneath the skin, we do not recommend this for home use. Such tumors are often enmeshed with blood vessels that may have to be surgically separated when the mass is ready to be expelled by the body. And separate it does, often to the absolute amazement of those who have never seen such a miracle! Our patients are tremendously pleased.

Supportive Products - Our recently developed ozone salve is an ideal companion product for the escharotic salve since it can be applied to the cavity and speed up the healing considerably. Chemically-bonded stable ozone, when applied to tissue, has unique oxygen donor properties conducive to a totally clean environment. Another companion product might be an ozone suppository which will increase the oxygen content of the blood considerably through the media of the rich bed of blood vessels in the lower bowel. This is a most welcome addition to our therapy which relies heavily on oxygen enhancement.

A prominent phyto (herb) chemist has also used the knowledge of how the escharotics work to develop formulations for internal use to assist in treating internal cancers. Several reports from satisfied consumers of these products indicate it is possible to remove cancer from inside the body as well as from the outside. We are presently testing these substances to see if they have a place in our therapy protocol. Preliminary results are very encouraging.

A Final Word

You have just concluded a comparatively non-technical, common-sense and clinically proven approach to a class of disorders that are epidemic in our nation today. You have the choice to agree with this program or you can continue to follow the edicts of the "school medicine" approach which tends to allow conditions to reach critical proportions before treatment is initiated.

Although our philosophy is firmly entrenched in the belief that health is our greatest wealth, it is quite sad for us to see how many quantify their treatment approach by dollars - "How much does it cost?" Ask any sick rich man what he would pay to have exuberant good health and you know what the answer would be. When you have health, you have everything.

Taking your health problem (large as it may seem) and breaking it down into smaller, treatable entities can only mean that you will improve. Building up the parts will inevitably result in a healthier whole. So go for it!

The Authors

WELCOME TO
HOSPITAL
SANTA MONICA

A Member Of The
Drs. Donsbach and Alsleben
Philosophy of Healing Care Centers
Institute Santa Monica - Poland
Health Restoration Institute - Tijuana
Hospital Santa Monica - Rosarito

These institutions are full care, well staffed and licensed facilities for the wholistic treatment of:
- **All types of Cancer**
- **Candidiasis & Chronic Fatigue**
- **Multiple Sclerosis**
- **Arthritis**
- **Heart Disease**
- **Stroke**
- **Detoxification Programs**

VIDEO CASSETTES AVAILABLE:
Cancer
Candidiasis/Chronic Fatigue
Cancer Testimonials
Health Through Detoxification

> **FOR MORE INFORMATION**
> **619-428-1146**

EMBRACING WHOLISTIC HEALTH

by Kurt W. Donsbach, D.C., N.D., Ph. D.

CLARIFYING THE
BODY - MIND - SPIRIT
CONNECTION
in
CANCER - ARTHRITIS - CANDIDIASIS
HEART DISEASE - MULTIPLE SCLEROSIS

Explicit treatment protocols from the world famous natural healing institutions - Hospital Santa Monica, Hospital St. Augustine and Institut Santa Monica

You can order this 300 page, profusely illustrated manual by checking with your local health food store or by calling 1-800-423-7662. Total cost - $14.95. Dr. Donsbach feels this is his best work yet. You should have this book on your shelf to help you answer health questions that may come up. It is the best review of the application and merits of wholistic health philosophy available today.